Sara's Story

Sara's Story

Multiple Sclerosis, Karmic Memories,
and the Good Doctor

Sara Willis

With a Medical Epilogue
by Wayne P. London, M.D.

Published in the USA by

Railroad Street Press
St. Johnsbury, VT
www.railroadstreetpress.com

Sara's Story:
Multiple Sclerosis, Karmic Memories and the Good Doctor.
    90 pp.   20 cm.
    ISBN 978-0-9844-7380-9
    Library of Congress Catalogue Number 2010902394
    1. Biography   2. Health   3. Spirituality
    BIO   2010
First Printing

CONTENTS

1 - From the start

I don't remember ever not seeing them; they fit so seamlessly into my life. Fortunately, my mother had a deep appreciation for imagination ... and later, for belief.

I never knew their first names, but that never mattered. I knew them as the Jenks family — mother, father, two boys and a girl. The children were close to my own age. And although I loved to play out of doors more than in, it was only inside that I saw them. At the time, it did not seem strange to me that their clothes were very different from what I or my parents wore.

We lived in a house with three apartments. Our home was on the first floor and consisted of two bedrooms, a kitchen, living room, and the schoolroom. My mother ran a private kindergarten in the 1950's - public schooling did not begin until first grade.

The kindergarten was opened when I was around five, and the schoolroom was originally the dining room; but the Jenkses were around even then.

The mother and father never spoke to me; just watched over us as we played. Certainly that was not unusual to me — it was what adults did. Besides, I was busy talking to the children and had no need for conversation with their parents.

We played mostly on the floor in the schoolroom with the toys from shelves which lined the walls; but if I went into the living room, they went with me.

The Jenks children sometimes even joined me at the table for a meal, although my mother did not serve them, or, in fact, even see them. But she trusted me, believed in me, even when I was that young, and she would ask, "Sara, were the Jenkses here today?" And if I said that yes, they were, she would ask what we had done. At first, she played along to encourage the creativity of make-believe; but, eventually, she came to believe I could see what she could not. It may have been that acceptance—her unfailing faith in me—which kept the door open between the spiritual realm and this one, the one many people believe is the only one. But there are those who do believe in that other realm, and a few who say that every child "sees" and is forced to stop seeing by adults determined to teach right from wrong, truth from lie. Punished for being far too imaginative—or for "fibbing"—most children quickly learn to see only what is considered real by the adults around them. I, on the other hand, was encouraged rather than discouraged by both my mother and my grandmother.

I was an outgoing child, sweet and chatty, and free to wander our small neighborhood; and so I went easily from house to house. I spoke in a way which, I am told, went far beyond my age, and some were quite taken by a tiny girl who acted like a very old soul. And if wisdom shows in a compassionate nature and in the ability to empathize, then perhaps that was one way I gained my reputation. I could not bear the cruel teasing of anyone; could not, especially, endure poor children being taunted or slow children being laughed at. And when I was old enough to go to school, what I saw and heard sometimes broke my heart.

I remember a little boy who was burdened not only by

his tattered clothes, but also by a terrible stutter. It was bad enough that the other children were merciless in their teasing, but even worse that the teacher did nothing to stop it. Outraged, I thought to myself, "I don't like this! What kind of a place is this? Get me out of here!" I simply could not understand the carelessness of those without kindness.

So, my world enlarged after I started first grade; some changes being good and some assuredly not so good. And although I continued to have experiences which were unusual, to say the least, my earliest encounter with spirits came to an end. The Jenks family went away, never to be seen or heard from again.

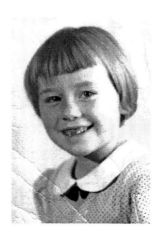

2 - Guidance from beyond

Several significant changes took place around the age of nine. It was then when I began to see beneath the superficial social behavior of others. I knew who was telling the truth and, often, who was not; I knew who could be trusted and who could not; I even knew, at times, who had been especially "bad".

Also, I began to hear conversations which were not loud enough to understand, as though a radio had been turned on with the volume left low.

But the most important, I believe, was the arrival of two women in my life—or perhaps I should say the spirits of two women. They visited three or four times each summer, returning regularly until I was eleven or twelve, and only occasionally after that. They wore skirts in bright colors, and their features were Native American. They appeared in my backyard, and I accepted their presence just as I had accepted the Jenks family. They spent their time advising me on how I should conduct myself, and they made it very clear that I must never let a lie pass my lips; that I should be kind and caring. They warned me about the dangers of excessive drinking and were adamant that I not be sexually active until marriage. The effect they had on me proved to be profound, for they set me on the path I would follow.

I ran everywhere as a child; I lived to run. I tore my friends away from dolls and indoor play. I convinced them to come outside, run through the woods; jump the brook.

But they never liked it the way I did.

I challenged myself to increase my speed, to compete with everyone and, most important of all, to win. Only one boy could beat me. I was the wind. I was Apache.

When the ladies in colorful skirts told me about Geronimo, somehow I already knew him. I could not watch Westerns on television because my connection was to the Indians, not the cowboys. And as I learned more, I was not merely sympathetic; I was outraged.

The Vietnam War was building when I was in high school, and my father supported our government's involvement. I shifted my hawkish stand on the plight of the Indian onto the plight of the American soldiers. I told myself I would join the Army, go to Vietnam and help in the cause. As a girl, I knew the only way to get there was to become a nurse. I plotted my future by planning the quick route to qualify: I would become a licensed practical nurse, even though I would have much preferred soldiering and carrying a rifle and engaging the enemy - becoming a warrior.

My father had no sons; but he had me - a daughter who, at the age of sixteen, loved to hunt. Through St. Johnsbury Academy, I took rifle lessons at the armory. Very much in my element, I also learned to use a handgun and became an excellent shot.

The warrior mentality was deeply ingrained long before I ever heard of Vietnam; but by the time the war was a nightly media event, my father was proud that I marched for the war, not against it.

I strengthened my moral code. By being truthful, I

believed that I could emulate Geronimo, who was known to always be truthful no matter the repeated betrayals by the American government. What I knew of Geronimo came from my guides, not from books.

It angered me that the Indians had receded beyond the Mississippi River. I wished they had taken a stand there, shooting all trespassers. And I felt justified by such thoughts.

It may seem contradictory that I condemned what had been done to the Native Americans by the same government which I now supported as it warred against the Vietnamese. But I was still a child with limited understanding; and perhaps what drove me most of all was an affinity for the soldiers themselves. To me, they were the warriors of my tribe; my people. And, as a matter of fact, there was one particular soldier who mattered to me most of all.

My cousin, Greg, was going to Vietnam; and I knew that I would be there with him.

He and I were only months apart in age, and I had always enjoyed his company immensely. He lived in New Hampshire; but whenever I visited, we had the best of times. Even during our teenage years, we could talk for hours. We even talked about reincarnation and war, but we never talked about him going to war, although I already had the "knowing" that he would be sent to Vietnam. And when the time came to say good-bye, I blocked out what I did not want to know about the future and about how his tour of duty might impact his life, changing him forever.

In 1969, a few short months before I would marry at the

age of twenty-two, I had a vision unlike any I had had before. I was in my room in my parents' house, staring at the aquarium as the fish swam round and round when I fell into a meditative state … and found myself beside my cousin, Greg. All sense of time vanished, and I saw Greg wounded and lying on the ground. I bent down, kissed him on the cheek and said, "I'll see you." I had no fear, no worry, but I heard the sounds of battle going on around us. And then I was back in my room, watching the fish.

I told no one about my vision.

Soon after this had happened, I came home one evening only to have my mother meet me at the door in a state of great upset. "Greg's been wounded!" she cried, alarmed nearly as much over how I would take it as she herself was over the terrible news. She knew how close we were.

I astounded her with my calm and reassuring response. "Don't worry," I said. "He'll be fine. We'll see him soon."

And we did. He recovered from his wounds and eventually worked for the Border Patrol at the Texas/Mexico border.

Apparently our psychic connection worked both ways, because he made reference once to my being with him at that terrible moment; and quite a few years later, he surprised his wife one day by suddenly blurting out, "Something special has happened to Sara. We have to call her."

Special, indeed! A second child had arrived—a beautiful baby girl, whom we named Kristal.

3 - Resolve and a prophesy

Since I choose to see life as a spiritual journey, then I know I must accept personal responsibility for the quality of my life. Obviously easier said than done; and I remind myself that it is a never-ending process.

I always believed in an afterlife. After all, it would have been hard not to believe when I'd always seen ghosts. And although some people might argue that what I thought I saw was not proof of life after death, for me there was never any doubt. I saw (and still see) people who once lived but no longer do.

They showed up unexpectedly. Sometimes they came along with my flesh and blood visitors. But, for the most part, there were no actual messages until later in my life. Or, perhaps, there were always messages and I simply did not feel my life would allow for opening up to them. I suppose it was all about belief—society's belief—and I certainly did not want to embarrass my family by going public with my psychic sensing.

I have never been afraid. Startled, yes; but afraid, no. At least, not of spirits.

I don't expect to convince those who cannot believe. But if I can give hope to those who are bereaved, if I can help bring closure to those who need answers, then that is reason enough to finally talk freely about it.

Because of my experiences, I have a great deal of faith; but that does not mean I am immune to frustration and disappointment. I still strive to let go of expectations, perhaps more than most people. After all, I sometimes have the inside track on what will probably happen, and I feel a strong desire to share that information. I understand that I cannot fix other's lives however much I may wish to help; but I must confess to sometimes meddling in what is none of my business, particularly when it comes to romance. I fancy myself a matchmaker, although I am none too successful at it. Sometimes I wish everyone would just follow my advice, so certain I am of my wisdom. But life has a way of putting me in my place, even though I sometimes have the ability to see and hear what others cannot.

I used to walk the two miles home from school each day, and it was an easy walk, until I was fifteen. Suddenly, in the month of May, I had to stop, not once, but again and again. I sat right down in the street, because I was too weak to walk continually. After each stop, I gathered myself together and through sheer force of will made my way home.

I told no one. Not my parents; not my friends. And two weeks later, the episodes of weakness passed as mysteriously as they had appeared. I did wonder what had happened to me, but I was not afraid. My not telling had nothing to do with fear; it had to do with my determination to be strong and capable.

A year passed. I was sixteen, already accomplished with a bow and arrow and discovering the thrill of shooting and hunting; and I was still running, if not as fast. And then it happened again — the weakness. This time, the attack was worse than the first. Still, I told no one. I managed to bluff my way through the two weeks; but I was very disturbed by what was happening to my body. I talked sternly to my legs. Their refusal to cooperate was completely unacceptable to me.

I used the time to sit under a tree on the hillside and think. I thought about so many things ... and I began to wonder about karma. I already believed in reincarnation. I'm not sure why. Certainly my parents had no such belief. But it made sense to me.

I thought about my "condition" and wondered if reincarnation played a part. And then I thought about my sense of connection to the Apaches. Had I lived a life as an Indian? Was that the origin of my deepening anger over their treatment?

Once again, the attack of weakness passed; but I was not back to normal. I could go to school, and I could walk, even run, but I was definitely not what I had been. And one glaring difference was that I could no longer play basketball. Neither was I winning at badminton the way I used to. My coordination had diminished significantly.

The following fall, it hit me again. It was November — hunting season — and I went into the forest on Monadnock Mountain with my father. I couldn't keep up. I kept falling — even my vision was affected - and I had no choice but to finally admit what had been happening to me.

I was taken to a doctor to be examined, but my parents kept the diagnosis to themselves. They must have been alarmed by the choices I later heard they were given: that it was either a brain tumor or multiple sclerosis.

The attack passed, but I was definitely the worse for wear. Still, I didn't despair. I would deal with whatever came at me. If I had to work harder and be stronger to fulfill my ambition, so be it.

My positive attitude may have been a boon for my mind, but it did not stop the ravaging of my body. In the spring of my senior year in high school, I had another attack; and this time it was horrendous. It affected more than my legs; it affected by bladder and bowels and led to humiliation in school. I wasn't a small child having an understandable accident. And though I cared little about the opinions of others, I did care about simple human dignity and normal privacy. Even so, I forced myself to push aside my embarrassment and return to school.

I turned eighteen on May 23, 1965, and I was clearly getting worse. I went into the hospital, and my doctor finally told me I had multiple sclerosis. I wasn't surprised, because a year and a half before this definite diagnosis, a classmate had asked me, "What's up? You always used to win at badminton, and now you only lose." For some unknown reason, I quickly replied, "It's because I have M.S."

During my stay in the hospital, I made a resolution. I would "do good" by cheering up others. I convinced my parents to bring me what I needed to make small gift baskets, and I took these around to other patients. It gave me a purpose. And I told God that if I could just keep going, keep walking, I would never stop trying to help others; never stop looking for those to whom I could bring a little happiness.

While I was in the hospital, I had a vision. It wasn't really a dream — although I cannot swear as to whether I was awake or asleep. However it came to me, it proved to be prophetic.

I was told that someday I would meet a doctor with black hair. Well, that certainly got my attention since my romantic notions always involved black-haired boys! This unnamed doctor would come to me - not the other way around - and his interest would be in the immune system, Multiple Sclerosis, and me as a person having paranormal experiences. I knew I was not to dwell on this future event, and I did not know when it would happen; but I was well aware of the importance of our meeting. It gave me hope for the future. I trusted the vision; and my attitude became "whatever will be, will be."

The first time I was given prednisone was during my stay in the hospital, and its effect was nearly miraculous. Back on my feet, I knew my life would be more challenging than I had once supposed; but I wasn't bitter. And I wasn't deterred. I set my sights on becoming a nurse, and I still believed I would join the Army.

4 - Spirits of the land

While I was in high school, my Native American mentors came to me once a year. But, for the most part, I was on my own. I spent a lot of my time thinking and trying to understand the world in which I lived. During those years of adolescence, there was a heightening of my ability to intuitively determine the true character of those with whom I came in close contact.

It was not easy being aware of the secrets adults might keep; and it was downright disturbing to "know" a much-admired man everyone fawned over was actually an adulterous spouse. I kept that sort of knowing to myself. But when friends wished for truthful opinions about hairstyles and clothing, I was the one they asked. And although I could not lie, I did learn to be diplomatic!

For the most part, I was exceedingly careful to keep my thoughts, feelings and experiences to myself. I did not wish to be the topic of gossip. Unfortunately, at a young age I already knew that few people were entirely trustworthy. Gossip is sometimes simple entertainment for someone's boring life, but it can also have a more devious purpose. Understanding the psychology which drives others to criticize and condemn only strengthens my commitment to work towards being non-judgmental myself, for I believe it is the cornerstone of a spiritual life.

I don't know when I began to realize there was a real confusion in my approach to life. On the one hand I was compassionate, understanding, and striving to evolve in a spiritually-positive way, while on the other hand I was fiercely committed to seeing justice done, even if it took violence to accomplish it.

It didn't make sense.

Unless, that is, I examined reincarnation more thoroughly.

There was a story—or, rather, part of a story—which kept coming back to me. Visions and vivid dreams have always been normal to me, and in this vision, this story, there was a room painted a certain shade of green (a color I would detest for the rest of my life). I saw teenage girls with long, shimmering black hair, and it seemed to me that I must have once actually been there in that room and that I must have once known these girls; and yet I knew that wasn't possible. None of my friends resembled these girls with oriental features. And although there was a negative energy attached to the room, there was also a sense of security; a sense of being warm, protected from the elements, of good food and a full belly.

When I first began to "see" this room, I did not understand why the girls paraded themselves by walking around the room. But, at the same time, I had the weirdest sense of wishing I could be the chosen one; the desired one.

It would be many years before the entire picture would emerge, but the sense of competition stayed with me always. There was also something connected to this "story" which somehow managed to bury itself in my subconscious, for I had very peculiar thoughts about the "fast" girls in my high school. I often wondered why they were willing to give away their value for nothing in return. Now, of course, I realize that these thoughts came from a past life, not this present one.

Something else from that past life seems to have affected me in this life. I love to barter! If a friend complains of having an abundance of cabbages in her garden the year I have an abundance of carrots, I'm quick to want to make an exchange - even though I can well afford to buy my cabbages at the store! But on a more serious note, I have had a vision of that life, and it was nothing to laugh at. I've seen myself, with a baby on my hip, bartering on the street, trying to survive.

I began the training to become a nurse, although it was obvious my health was now an obstacle. And it wasn't long before I had to confront the obvious—the Army would never take me. Desperate, I toyed with the idea of offering my future nursing services to The Good Ship Hope. I wanted—I needed—to find something worth fighting for.

But the war I was to fight would involve only me. There would be no heroics, no battlefield injuries to tend to; no historic struggle fighting for freedom. My great war would ultimately be with Multiple Sclerosis.

Only three months into the nursing program, I dropped out and went home.

Our family owned a shoe store, and I had worked there summers helping out. Now, it was where I would find my only employment; and I rose to the challenge. I'm proud of that, because sometimes the most difficult challenge is in giving up the grand plan in favor of the simple.

I found it easy and enjoyable to talk to people; and I absolutely loved selling. So I did my best to move forward with my life. Even if nursing was out of the picture, I could still be helpful.

As an adult, I found a kind of normalcy by living and working in a small town. I went out on dates; even dated a young man who had been in the Air Force. I learned (only after he was gone) that he was a full-blooded Chiricahua, a tribal group of the Apache. It is interesting to me that what I thought was simple attraction to boys with black hair may well have been, instead, a past-life memory.

When he moved back home to Ohio, I was lonely enough that my friend, Carol, suggested I go out on a double date with her, her boyfriend, and a college student whose name was David.

Just for fun, I had my palm read on the Thursday before my planned first date with David. (For some reason, it's much easier for me to receive clear information about everyone else!) Still, I wasn't really expecting anything earth-shattering, and what I heard that day could only be proven with time.

The woman had three important things to tell me. The first was that my disease would not get the best of me. While that may have been something I wanted to hear, it wasn't a surprise. Not to me. I was already aware of how stubborn I could be in the face of difficulties.

The second thing she told me was that although I would have children, I would choose not to give birth. Again, not a big surprise. I'd never been one to moon over the idea of childbirth; and, of course, there was the health consideration. But I did want to be a mother.

And then she told me that the man I was about to go out with on Saturday night would want to marry me ... although she seemed to have no ability to foretell my feelings toward him!

Looking back, my encounter with the palm reader gives me a good chuckle. Forty years later, I'm still walking (aided by canes and a walker), and I'm enjoying my life; my adopted children are grown and have given me grandchildren; and last, but not least, I remain very much married to David.

What she didn't tell me were all the other details which make up a life - the joys and heartaches, the times of struggle and the times of ease, the worry and the fretting, and the learning to let go. She never mentioned the exciting times which lay ahead, or the disappointing times. She didn't say how hard life could be … or how magical. And I'm glad she wasn't able to tell me, because those were the things I wanted to discover on my own — either through intuition or experience.

I have always been thrilled that I often "get" information. I find it amazing that the future is there for the reading; that I can sit quietly, ask a question and receive the answer. It is reassuring when what I "get" proves true, because it means I have not been imagining it. But when that truth is sad, or even tragic, I might wish it had been only my imagination. It's not easy realizing that someone has little time left in this life, especially when I'm the only one who realizes it.

6 - Our family

Early in our marriage, the place David and I lived in had a garage beneath the house, and we accessed it by going down the basement stairs.

One morning, after David had left for work, I heard the sound of someone walking in the street outside our window. The steep embankment across the street prevented building there, so it was a street with very few houses, and it was rare to hear anyone nearby.

When I heard footsteps coming up the stairs from our garage, I was shocked that an intruder had somehow gotten into the house; and I did exactly what every scary movie loves to show us: I actually opened the door at the top of the stairs!

But unlike the scary movies, there was no one there.

This all happened shortly after a horrific crime had been committed in Chicago and gained national attention. Overnight, I (and probably every other young woman in America) had become extremely fearful. For that reason, my focus that day was on living, breathing threats, and my heart was pounding when I opened the door.

David's father had passed away only one month before, and I was certain, as I looked down the empty staircase, that it was he who had knocked. Unfortunately, distracted by my fear of the living, and not yet having learned how to ask outright for any messages a spirit might bring, I said nothing. Perhaps if I had, my father-in-law might have been able to communicate further with me, either by showing me his spirit or by impressing upon me what it was he had come to say. Instead, it was simply a lost opportunity.

After only one year in our first house, we moved to another, right next door to my parents. It would be our home for three years.

My mother was diagnosed with cancer while we lived there, and we all understood that she was dying. She and I even talked about how she might be able to communicate with me after she passed over. The plan was for her to move my plants around — probably not the best idea, since it must take an enormous amount of energy for a spirit to manipulate objects.

As it turned out, after she died, the only thing out of the ordinary was loud whistling coming from the basement when no one but me was around to hear it.

During the time we lived in that house, my sense of knowing grew increasingly stronger. I often had a sense of what was going to happen - and one of the best things to happen was a little boy coming into our lives. My beloved mother had died, but now I was to be a mother myself.

Steven arrived at the age of two, and he was a delight.

7 - Being psychically sensitive

We made plans to move again. This time, it would be to an old farmhouse which had been in my husband's family since the 1700's. Round Barn Farm was a wonderful place. Its mowed fields stretched out gracefully to the banks of the Passumpsic River, and Joe's Brook tumbled ferociously down the mountainside across the road to join with the Passumpsic and then flow into the Connecticut River.

Just before we moved there in 1975, David's aunt and uncle still lived in the house; but whenever we visited them, I liked sitting outside on a large rock near the garden, getting a feel for the place.

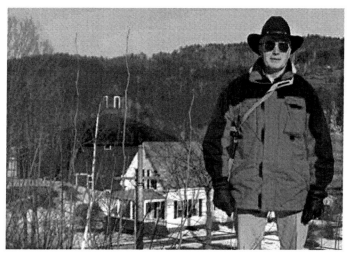

David at Round Barn Farm

From the beginning, I saw spirits there. At first, as I sat on the rock, gazing out across the lowest land which the river sometimes flooded into, I saw a young Native American man in a canoe. Sometimes, I saw him walking along the bank. And then, after we moved into the farmhouse and my own life became full and rich with family and accumulated years, what I was seeing on a spirit plane also evolved and broadened. Eventually, I saw others going about their daily routines; and I continued to watch that same man as he matured, courted a young woman and swam with her in the river. At some point, I realized they had married, and over the years, that they had produced three children.

There were so many others, coming and going — even climbing to the ledges of the mountain. I sensed their presence everywhere around the farm and surrounding area.

But I needed quiet in order to move into that place where time and space shifted for me so that I could be an observer of what had once thrived on the Passumpsic long before I moved to Round Barn Farm; long before I was even alive. When my children were old enough to go to school, I had more time to sit on the back porch, to meditate and pray; and I opened even more to whatever this ability was that I was born with.

I rarely spoke of what I saw. I was well aware that others found it difficult, even impossible, to believe I was in my right mind. Even today, when there is enough interest to warrant movies and television shows which showcase psychically sensitive characters, I understand that what I report will be questioned. I don't know why some of what I see is symbolic and some is real, why some messages are clear and others are hard to interpret. But the Universe speaks to me in its own language.

There was a bedroom in the farmhouse where I always felt a presence; and I remember that I also sensed that same presence frequently in the living room. It would arrive on a whiff of potent barn odor. The scent of manure, when there had been no cows on the farm for many years, would have been enough to grab anyone's attention! I would look up, and although I saw nothing, I would imagine a farmer coming into the room and sitting in the chair which was placed in the corner by the doorway leading to the kitchen.

Once, (and this is one of the wildest things I've seen!) I went outside to drive a babysitter home. It was dark, but I could still see well enough. A man was in the yard, dressed all in black; and although he wore a hat, he had no head! I could see clear through that space between hat and cloak. I noticed that the dogs saw him, too; and I wondered why they didn't bark as they always did at strangers. Instead, they seemed quite comfortable with him. But I, unlike the dogs, ignored him and went on my way, and I never saw him again. If he had a message, I have no idea what it might have been.

There was a piece of land across the road which was a part of the farm. It was wooded, except for a small area which we kept clear. Although it was close by the road, because of the woods, it was well-hidden. It was (and is) a place energized by the rapidly-flowing waters of Joe's Brook and, I believe, by the people who once lived there. There was a one-time visitor to the farm who, apparently, also had abilities outside of the norm; and she told me that when she walked up into that spot, she saw children running through a small village, as well as other signs of Indian life. Although I did not see specifically what she saw, I certainly sensed it, and I have always been drawn to the place. Today, it is where I live in a new house, and where I keep a labyrinth. It is a place for meditation and contemplation; a place to connect with nature. It is a spiritual place of healing energy.

I wanted to give my children a fanciful explanation for the unexplainable because I did not want them to be fearful. Strange sounds, especially in the night, are not always from the normal creaks and groans of an old house. The wind isn't always blowing, the furnace isn't always running. And so I told them that all over the world there were little people living in the fields and woods who sometimes entered houses without anyone seeing. Although these little people were mischievous, they caused no harm. They liked to hide things just to enjoy our frustration as we searched for what we thought we had lost. These little people were known by many names, but we would call them by their Irish name—leprechauns. My children could not see what I was seeing, but they could hear.

At the risk of sounding too fanciful myself, I will share this seemingly storybook tale:

One day, while sitting on the porch, I noticed one of my Native American ladies standing on the walk. I hadn't seen my mentors in quite a few years, and so I was surprised—but not nearly as surprised as I soon would be.

As its name implies, Round Barn Farm has one of the few remaining barns built using a circular design. The distance from the back porch of the house to the barn is not far, and another barn sits close to it. But there is a wide swath of ground which runs between the barns and the house. It is a gentle slope through the fields down to the

Passumpsic River, but it is intersected by railroad tracks.

That day, as I sat on the porch, a movement caught my eye, and when I looked, there came down the tracks what, at first, I thought was a Palomino horse, but smaller — more the size of a Welsh pony. Then I noticed that a horn grew from his forehead. Now, I realize that a unicorn is considered a mythological creature, but I could not deny that I did indeed see a horn!

He left the tracks and pranced into our meadow, stopping now and then to nibble on the grass; and he remained there, grazing and prancing, for several hours. Even after I had gone into the house to tend to my chores, I checked periodically, and he was still there.

During those hours, I also noticed that both of my Indian guides were standing in the doorway of the round barn, talking to each other. Although they said nothing to me, it was obvious that they were aware of my presence; and when they finally left, I again watched the goings-on in the meadow, and I saw the man from the canoe jump onto the unicorn's back and ride away to the south.

Clearly, there must have been a message in this strange happening; but as with the most puzzling of dreams, I cannot interpret it to this day.

I am not afraid of spirits, but I do have a healthy fear of people breaking into the house, especially while I am sleeping. And since I have always heard footsteps on the stairs, I have also always had my share of adrenaline-pumped scares while I wait to discover if the sounds are coming from someone in this world or not!

One night, getting up to use the bathroom, I encountered a woman standing in the hallway. She certainly startled me, but since she said nothing, I managed to pass her by without any comment of my own.

There were other instances where I sensed the spirits of the departed in and around the house — women sitting in the TV room, the farmer, the Native Americans. But, for the most part, there was no communication - just my own wondering.

One exception happened when my daughter, Kristal, was fifteen years old. She was friends with a talented, athletic girl who had been diagnosed with a heart abnormality which, it was thought, had been corrected when she was very young. Unfortunately, one fateful day she collapsed as she walked into school, and later died from a heart attack.

Less than six months after her tragic and unexpected death, she came to me with a message for her parents. I vividly remember the Red Sox baseball cap she was wearing at the time, and it was that hat which helped me to recognize her. She had been a huge Red Sox fan and had enjoyed her trips to Fenway Park to watch them play.

I was lying awake in my bed when I saw her and she spoke to me; and I was later very relieved that her parents were open to what I had to tell them. It felt wonderful to be able to bring a measure of comfort in the midst of their grieving.

A few years later, a spirit encounter set in motion a life-changing event in my own life. It was early one morning, and David was in the shower while I lay in bed, slowly waking to the day. A young man was standing at the foot of the bed. I should have been shocked, but I wasn't (which is always a clue that it's a spirit); and I listened to him explain that he had committed suicide. Disturbing, yes ...and yet he also said, "I want to tell you that my grandfather and I have had a wonderful time today fishing Joe's Brook!" He then gave me a message for his mother, who worked for The American Society of Dowers in Danville, Vermont—fortunate for me since dowsers are well-known for having open minds when it comes to such matters as messages from the spirit world!

And it was through this woman that the vision I'd seen so many years before would finally become a fulfilled prophecy. I was about to meet a doctor who would present me with a whole new theory on healing.

9 - Descent

Throughout the child-rearing years, my condition steadily worsened. I was always tired, my legs grew weaker, and I needed to spend more and more time resting.

Another difficulty arose which I did not understand at the time was part of my disease. I suffered from inappropriate laughter, as well as inappropriate tears. It seemed my emotions had their wires crossed. I worried constantly that I would upset others and embarrass myself, and so I had no choice but to use extreme care about the places I went.

Our son was in a terrible automobile accident; and although we counted our blessings when he healed against all odds, we still had to deal with the subsequent court case. Out-of-control laughter in such a serious setting would probably unnerve anyone. But for me, married to an attorney, such behavior was mortifying. Bad enough that I embarrass myself, but absolutely devastating to me that I should embarrass my dignified husband.

By the time the 1990s rolled around, I could no longer walk in the woods. I mourned over the loss of something which had always been vital to my emotional well-being. The numbness in my feet became an advancing army slowly creeping up my legs. My entire right leg and my left leg as far as the knee were dead to sensation. It was like trying to walk around on wooden stilts. I had no idea if my feet were cold; and living in a northern climate, this created a very real concern. Even my "plumbing" was betraying me. I could not recognize the sensation of needing to urinate, and by 1995, I had barely one-third bladder control remaining.

Just as disturbing to me was the fact that I was obviously suffering what I considered to be mental confusion. I, who had once been agile and athletic, who had been well-coordinated and an expert marksman couldn't even figure out how to reach out and catch a set of tossed car keys. Of course, what was actually happening was that the myelin covering on my nerves — my insulation — was being destroyed, and the "instant messaging" normal brains are capable of engaging in, in order to communicate with the body, was not available to my forlorn brain.

At the age of forty-seven, determined though I had always been, even I could see the writing on the wall.

Through the years, many suggestions had been made about which medications or treatments might be advantageous. The ones I tried did not help; and those I refused to try didn't appear to be helping anyone else suffering from multiple sclerosis, so I chose not to impoverish my family by paying exorbitant sums for false cures. I attended a support group where new medications were discussed; but I never saw anyone there improving. My husband would have paid any price to help me heal, but I already knew that what was being offered through traditional medicine would not help me.

10 - It's how you play the game

When I was growing up, obedience was expected from children. Talking back, as they called it, was not well tolerated, and the giving of praise was stingy at best. My sister was born when I was three years old, and I always felt the added pressure of being the oldest child. I loved both my parents, and I knew they loved me; but as I grew, I learned to keep my opinions to myself. I bottled up my feelings so expertly that I ceased to cry. Unfortunately, I also nearly ceased to laugh.

There was a man by the name of John who lived next door to us when I had just begun my teens. He was only a bit more than a decade older, but twenty-six was a grown-up to me. He was incredibly kind—willing to play badminton and even give me a ride on his motorcycle; and he talked to me in a way that was never inattentive or condescending.

I remember one day when he spoke up to my father with some exasperation. I don't remember what my father had reprimanded me for, but I will never forget the words John spoke. "Can she never do anything right?"

John married and had a child, and I was happy to babysit - he and his family were very important to me. But, like my cousin Greg, John ended up in Vietnam; and though he wrote, when his tour of duty ended, his family had moved away and he never came to visit us again. After all these years, I can still feel how much it mattered to have his attention, his caring, and his kindness -

especially at a time in my life when, like all girls that age, I craved some reassurance from a male that I was worth spending time with. How fortunate for me that what I received from John was exactly what I needed, and it was given in a safe and appropriate manner.

When John heard about my being diagnosed with Multiple Sclerosis, he wrote to me. And in that letter, he quoted the phrase everyone knows so well - though at the time I had never heard it. It's not whether you win or lose; it's how you play the game. This made a huge impression on me, and I would think of it many, many times over the years which followed.

Once I was diagnosed, my father never again had a harsh word for me — not even to this day.

11 - A healing feeling

When I was 48 years old, my life began to change in a way which would prove to be dramatic, although it started out simply enough.

I received a phone call from a man who said he was associated with The Dowsers' Society, and he asked for permission to visit me.

It was in the summer, and we sat on the screened porch. He was older than I, but his hair was still coal black. He was very nice, very caring, and we talked for a long time about all the things I would normally have been reticent to discuss — my disease, reincarnation, spirits, psychic messages — as well as life in general.

I learned he was a Harvard-educated psychiatrist; and although he had, until then, worked traditionally, he was interested in the role past lives might play in the occurrence of disease (not merely through karmic influence, but also genetically). He had a real appreciation for the metaphysical/spiritual approach to disease — an approach he found sorely lacking in Western medicine. During the many visits which followed that first visit, I would hear from him about the spiritual healing rituals of Native Americans. He would talk about mythologies and the use of the serpent to represent that which needed healing; about nature, the earth and its flowing waters, about dance, music, song and chanting being the tools through which healing could be drawn; that a surge of energy would follow such healing, leading to renewal, rebirth - a new way of being in this world.

But on that first day when our visit came to an end, I knew only that when he gave me a hug, I immediately felt a strong, intuitive sense of connection. After he left, I wondered if he was the one in my vision from thirty years before; but I didn't wonder for long. He scheduled visits on a regular basis; and the more we talked, the more my world began to shift. Until then, I had found my strength in the idea John had given me when I was first diagnosed—it's how you play the game—and for me, that was about keeping a stiff upper lip and accepting the way things were.

I did not understand the entire complex theory that Dr. Wayne London would present to me over the following several years, but I understood this: that "warrior" memories (feelings of anger and a desire for revenge) might cause disease; and that the memories did not have to necessarily mean one had actually lived a particular past life. Certainly I had always been fiercely attached to the Geronimo story, to the injustice perpetrated upon the Native Americans; and if that attachment was contributing to my illness, I needed to find a way to release it.

With Dr. London's help, I examined my life.

Part of Dr. London's theory is the belief that two of the major categories that diseases fall into are: auto-immune diseases (overactive immune system) such as multiple sclerosis, rheumatoid arthritis, lupus, and type 1 diabetes (marked by having something in one's life that does not belong), and immune-suppression diseases such as AIDS, viruses, and cancers (marked by the need for something which is missing in one's life). I'm glad I had the courage to look at how this might translate for my own situation, and it was soon obvious to me that my focus on Indian injustice — my intense anger at that injustice — was the something which did not belong in my life.

At Dr. London's suggestion I eventually began to read as much as I could about the historical Geronimo and the Native American struggle to survive; and over the course of three months, reading continuously, I cried continuously. Slowly, those tears began to cleanse me. Later, I would be curious enough to ask Dr. London more questions; but at the time, all that really mattered to me was that I was getting better. Feeling was returning to my legs, starting at the most far-away point — my big toe!

And none too soon was it happening, because by the time I met Dr. London, my condition had seriously deteriorated, and my fatigue was such that I needed long naps just to make it through the day. Bladder and bowel problems were worse; unexpected hysterical laughter made me so nervous that I chose to be housebound rather than risk losing control in public; and my mental confusion left me unable to even play with my grandchildren. When a ball was thrown my way, I sat with what must have been a dull expression. I couldn't think fast enough to respond with even that simple gesture of lifting my hand to catch a child's ball.

But my proper grieving — my three full months of weeping — allowed me to let go of the anger that did not belong. And in its place was room for the spiritual journey I would finally begin in order to find my authentic self.

12 - Past lives

I spent some time working with a man who used hypnosis to regress me. Although reincarnation was already an accepted belief for me, and I had my own memories which I attributed to past lives, I still found the regressions interesting.

During the sessions, I retrieved a life in Japan, and I felt the conviction that love for family and country was of the utmost importance; that pride and sacrifice were absolutes.

But probably the most significant life I remember is from 1400s England. I was a seamstress and a loving grandmother. My daughter came and went at will, leaving me with the responsibility of my beautiful small granddaughter. She was my very heart in that life, and that intense love is still with me. I know the identity of both daughter and grandchild, and they are with me in this life, too, although in different relationships (as well as form!). I find myself trying to reunite them still; and it makes both of them laugh. They tell me that my playing cupid is way off the mark. But I insist I'm right. They would be good together, are meant to be together; and I have often been frustrated by their resistance to my advice.

This is not the first time David and I have been together, whether he believes it or not. We, too, are meant to be together. We have work to do (a re-pairing for repairing). I love him dearly, and I know he loves me. I'm grateful he allows me to be who I am, but I wish he could believe as I do.

My memory of the Asian house of girls, I am certain, has influenced me in my life as Sara. I've always been strongly aware of my sexuality; and I'm fortunate that my spiritual guides impressed upon me the need for restraint in my behavior. What might have proven to be problematic was, instead, not a problem at all. But, luckily for me, David was my match in marriage, and that which I had held back since puberty could be expressed with him. But a certain hang-up which accompanied the vigilance over my virginity was the surprising criticism I felt toward those who were not acting "morally." This didn't fit with who I really am, since I have never felt I was better or worse than anyone else; and so I came to believe that the "criticism" was a holdover from that past life. Another possible hang-up was far from obvious back then, although it gives me pause to consider it now. The second chakra, located in the reproductive organs of the body, is the seat of sexuality and movement. My disease limited my movement. Might it also have been a way for me to limit my sexuality?

There are many questions unanswered. Have I created my disease? Did my soul come into this world with specific challenges in mind? And if that is true, it wouldn't be much of a test if the challenge could be easily overcome. So, did I choose my parents (and, therefore, my genetics, intelligence and socio-economic situation) in order to set up the life situations best suited for creating my challenges?

I try to see how my attitude, beliefs, expectations and needs create the life I'm now living. Even with my ever-growing understanding, I struggle to see myself clearly.

I also try to understand the way in which my soul may have created this life for me in order to make up for other lives. I know people who do not want to accept the kind of responsibility that this way of thinking suggests; but if it can be done without blame, without feeling as though I have somehow failed, then I can approach my life with excitement, humor and peace. Although some people may be presently experiencing their first incarnation, I believe many of us have lived before, many times; and that over the course of those lives we have experienced (and committed) just about everything. Karma is not punishment from a harsh God. It's simply a way for us to learn and evolve until we truly understand that we are not separate. We are connected. We are all one.

13 - Messages and mysteries

Starting in the 1990s, my paranormal experiences increased in number, and the receiving of specific messages became quite common for me. Prior to the nineties, it had been more about seeing and knowing.

I used to visit my uncle in the nursing home before he died, although he and my aunt (my mother's sister) had been divorced for many years. But after he passed, I saw him appear at my window at home - smiling and waving joyously (he'd always loved a good joke and plenty of laughter). He brought a substantial message for my aunt; and luckily for me, my aunt is a believer. I am not at liberty to reveal the message, but it had great meaning for her.

Once, a man from Danville simply appeared in my living room sitting on the couch. I recognized him immediately, because I had known him since I was a child. He had a message for his family, and I was relieved when the message was well-received. The only odd part about that visit was that Dr. London's father showed up at the same time, and the two men sat on my living room couch conversing for hours. I went about my business, but looked in from time to time, and they were still there. My thought at the time was that they had known each other in a past life. It was somewhat common for spirits to "hang out" for a while after giving me their messages, and so I did not find it strange that they spent the afternoon

Now, the reader might wonder why I didn't ask the two

men a lot of questions about what it was like on "the other side", but I took the burden of responsibility for listening to their messages very seriously. My concern was that I get their messages right so that I could pass along exactly what they had to say. And afterwards, I always found it taxing emotionally to make the appropriate phone calls. Whenever there was evidence of "proof", whenever the messages were received graciously, I sighed with relief.

During the years I lived at the farm, I sensed the constant presence of an old woman, although I have never seen her features clearly. She appears more as a silhouette. Her name is Hildegard, and I am well aware that she wants to help me, for I can "feel" her thoughts and her guidance. She has even gone, at my request, to help those I am especially worried about, although I realize she can only be a caring presence for them. However, for me, because I know she is there, I sometimes ask, "What should I do?", and that is when I hear her advice. Hildegard is, indeed, my spiritual guide.

Spirits are everywhere. They are around us all the time. They can be seen, heard, sensed … or ignored. But they are near us, not far - unless one considers a different dimension to be far away.

What I find frustrating are those times when I don't know how to act on a message which feels urgent. Many times I received the message that Dr. London needed to meet a man neither of us knew. I was given the man's name, but other than that, I was baffled … at least, for a while. Eventually, I learned who he was, and introductions were made, followed by many meetings where I was present. This man was quite ill, and though his body was not to heal, I believe he benefitted from knowing Dr. London. At one particular meeting where there were quite a few other people present, and in the middle of their discussion, I could see Native American spirits through the window. I said nothing, and it was obvious I was the only one seeing them; but at one point, three people mentioned they felt as though they had been touched on the back. The spirits simply wanted their presence recognized. Perhaps they had once known the man who was ill in another time. I can only get a sense, of course.

This same evening I had the opportunity to talk to the sick man's Uncle. He told me that recently when he was in California, he had seen young Apaches dance. This made me happy beyond what one can believe.

The next day, the last area which had remained numb between my left leg, knee and hip disappeared. Now there were no numb areas remaining in my body.

When David's mother died, she came to see me, insisting that my son was going to move next to a school. Although he lived in Burke at the time, I took this to mean that he should move to Concord right away because a house was for sale there with a very slight view of the school. Instead, he moved to another town where, by seeming coincidence, the house was right next to that town's school! But in trying to make the message fit the situation, I made the mistake of insisting he should immediately move to Concord. It taught me an important lesson: It's easy to misinterpret if I jump to conclusions. I was too attached to the outcome of the "message" I had received, and I tried to force it upon my son - perhaps to prove to myself that I had gotten it "right."

Sometimes, I see things which defy imagination. For instance, I once saw a thimble float down the stairs and across the room. I think I was too astounded to consider the possibility of a message attached to it. Perhaps it was simply a spirit moving about in her own world, and all I could see was the thimble on her finger.

One of my most astounding visions involved a battle which I believe took place during the French and Indian War. The vision unfolded as I lay in bed one night, and it prevented me from sleeping. It was not at all pleasant to see...or participate in! That's right—participate. I was there...and I was shot. And although I saw myself surviving the wound, many did not survive. Terrible things were done in that battle; and viewing it has left me with an indelible memory—much the same way a particularly gruesome and disturbing movie might leave me with a bad memory. I was able to identify many of the soldiers—both British and Colonist—as people I have known in this life. Interesting to me was how many of them, in this present-day life, have suffered from illnesses and tragedies (including myself). But once again, the karma is for the learning, not for the punishment. The opportunity to make amends gives joy to the soul. It feels good to help others. One man in particular, who distinguished himself in that battle, is the same man who has distinguished himself in business in this life. In battle, he was fearless, aggressive, and nearly indestructible ... just as he is now. But there are consequences to wartime acts (whether the war is deemed legitimate or not). Killing, in any form, has karma attached to it; and I know of some of the suffering this man has endured in this lifetime.

I don't know if everything which happens is meant to happen - but, for sure, some things are meant to happen. David and I were meant to live at Round Barn Farm. There is a connection for David which goes beyond family, although the family history is still an integral part of that connection.

John Russell, David's great, great uncle lived on the farm when the Civil War commenced in 1861. He went to Massachusetts to join up, probably because the enlistment bonus was greater than he would have gotten in northern Vermont; and that extra money would have greatly benefitted his family. While he was gone, his sister married a hired man by the name of Moore. And although John returned from the war, it is certain he was not unscathed by the terrible cruelties of war. He never married but worked alongside his brother-in-law, dying at a fairly young age. His sister and brother-in-law were to be David's great, great grandparents. David's uncle, Russell Moore, lived at Round Barn Farm with his wife when David and I married.

I believe the farmer I sometimes got a whiff of, fresh from the barn, was John Russell. After the Civil War, he had nowhere else to go but home; and after he died, he simply continued with his daily routine.

On one occasion, I had far more than a simple whiff of barn odors, and more than a quiet sense of his presence. It happened early one morning. At the time, I told myself I had gotten up to check on the cat (for what other possible reason could there have been for rising from bed while David still slept?). But now, years later, I realize I was drawn down the hall by some other force.

There, in another bedroom, in the middle of the bed and beneath the covers was an enormous lump. And it was moving. I wasn't afraid (which should have been a major clue!), and I didn't call out to David. As I watched, the lump continued moving ... until two feet (in boots, no less!) popped out from under the covers at the bottom of the bed, followed by the legs. Finally, the entire man appeared. He was wearing farmer's clothes, circa late 1800s; and he stood up.

I suspect we had similar expressions of interest as we stood looking directly at each other; and I noticed he had beautiful blue eyes. Finding my voice, I uttered the words, "My goodness! You must be John Russell!"

Whereby, he simply disappeared.

A particularly strange event happened some years ago. An elderly woman entered our glassed-in porch off the kitchen one evening. It was already dark, and certainly too cold for anyone to be wandering about. She was wearing a dress and dark coat and appeared a bit confused. Concerned, I asked where she lived. Her only response was, "From around here." David saw her, too, and he spoke to her, which led me to believe she was not one of my psychic visions, even though I did not feel alarmed the way I normally would have upon finding a complete stranger entering our house.

When she got up, insisting on leaving, we called the

State Police because we were worried about her safety; but they never found her. No one fitting her description was reported missing, and we did not see her again. David is certain she lived in this reality. But as for me? Well, it goes without saying that I believe she was a ghost.

14 - Karmic illness

Since coming to believe that uncovering someone's "story" (from a past life) is one of the keys to healing the present (as well as the past), I have had a few opportunities to work with those who are curious about, and at times anxious to use the information I receive intuitively. I believe such information can be used to improve their lives in the here and now.

I am well aware that many people cannot - or will not - accept the idea of having lived many lives. I know that there are those who find the idea of karma absurd, if not downright frightening. But if I did live before and did commit offenses - if I was a cruel master, a thief or a beggar, a saint or a sinner, if I was rich in one life and poor in another, if I was both loving and hateful, revengeful and forgiving, if I lived as a man, as a woman, as a black at one time, as red and then yellow before this life when I am white, if my lives sometimes ended in old age and sometimes as a newborn baby in my mother's arms, if I was at one time a killer and at another time the one being tragically killed, then it stands to reason that eventually my soul would be humbled enough to understand human failures, to have a great level of compassion for others, and to finally leave all judgment up to God.

Sometimes, all I need to do is meet someone and I begin "seeing" the story which is impacting his or her present life. But usually that happens only when I am specifically asked about someone; and that is when the flow of information is as clear as a movie playing in my mind. It may take only an instant, it may take hours, or it may take days for the full story to emerge. But I generally find myself caught up in the emotional drama. There are even times when I cannot sleep for all that is happening in my mind's eye.

Once, I met a man who also suffered from my affliction. He follows the traditional treatment for Multiple Sclerosis and is content for that to be his path toward healing as much as is possible in this life. But, in spite of his lack of interest in finding a physical healing through a metaphysical approach, he is still curious about past lives, and we have had the opportunity to sit and discuss his "story."

I saw him in a uniform, recognized him as Spanish, and I felt certain he had traveled from Mexico into what would become Texas, and then over into Florida. He was obviously in charge, and his brutality extended to his own men, not merely the natives he encountered. It was my sense that he was claiming land for Spain.

Centuries later, in this present life, he suffered abuse at the hands of his father during a difficult childhood. I do not see his disease as punishment for the past, but simply as an opportunity for his soul to learn. And perhaps his father offered up his own life in order to play the "bad guy" this time around in order to give his son the chance to experience being on the other side of brutality. Regardless, none of this means that it's all right to brutalize anyone. Of course it's not right! But it happens, and it will keep happening … unless and until we all evolve in our understanding that we are spiritual beings temporarily residing in a physical world; until we remember that we are all one, that our separateness is just a test, and that what we do to each other, we are doing to ourselves.

Cast your bread upon the water, and it will return to you many fold.

You reap what you sow.

What goes around comes around.

You get back what you give out.

Like begets like.

He who lives by the sword, dies by the sword.

Do unto others as you would have them do unto you.

Forgive us our trespasses as we forgive those who trespass against us.

And as Jesus also said: As you do unto the least of my brethren, you do also unto me.

There are probably a hundred ways of saying the same thing, and we've all heard it put one way or another - whether in church, from our mothers and fathers, from a thoughtful writer or speaker, or a wise friend - but apparently it bears repeating, over and over again, until we truly understand what it means. And although I come from a Christian background, the same directive can be found in other religions and other philosophies.

I've had spirits visit me, hang out with me, even ride in the car with me. I've been asked to deliver both simple messages and complicated messages; but, basically, what the dearly departed want their loved ones to know is I love you. And because of that, it may not look like proof of anything. But I feel the emotion behind the message; and love is the most powerfully satisfying emotion there is. When I receive a message, it comes through my heart, not my head — it comes with feeling.

15 - Native memories in OK and the West

I have a memory of an Indian village which existed in the latter half of the 1800s in what is now the State of Oklahoma. It was a time when most of the Native Americans had already been pushed west from their homes in the east, and the final destruction of Indian culture was fast approaching. Although Geronimo was not about to give up the fight, there were many Indians who understood that the only chance at survival for the people was to capitulate to the whites. Treaties were signed and broken; promises made and revoked. Small bands of angry warriors refused to follow their elders into surrender and, instead, went off on their own to continue the fight.

Although the tribe in this particular village was Lenni Lenape, also known as the Delaware Indians, connected to the Algonquin, they had been pushed out of their native lands (parts of the region now known as Delaware, Pennsylvania, New Jersey and New York). Lenape society was matriarchal (although there was a ruling Chief and a council of elders), and the women shared in decision-making. In the east, they had lived in longhouses in small villages and depended on corn, squash and beans. Lenni Lenape means true men or common people. They were peaceful, spiritual and just. And, in what proved to be their downfall, they were generous in their acceptance of the European settlers. When the Delaware were driven west to Oklahoma, they joined with Choctaw, Cheyenne, Seminole, and Iowa Indians.

Oklahoma territory was a very alien landscape after their agricultural lifestyle in the hills and the valleys of the east. Instead of enjoying a lush growing season, they were transplanted onto a flat, dry land where occasional torrential rains merely ran off the hard, cracked earth, forming dangerous rivers before disappearing as readily as they appeared, the land quickly returning to near desert.

I was Apache then, and at six years old, a chubby, happy, inquisitive child. Fascinated by the world around me, I often wandered about, playing and talking to myself, sometimes stopping to examine bugs.

A small band of Delaware Indians watched one day as I drifted away from my family's village on one of my excursions; and when the opportunity was ripe, they swept me away. A Lenape child had been lost, and this one was destined to take her place. Adopted into the family of a boy near my own age, I grew to love him ... but not before enduring the devastation caused by the loss of my own family. But the boy was always there to help as I slowly adjusted to my new home.

The grandmother of the family was a tribal elder with great influence, and she increasingly spoke of making peace with the whites. Years had passed, conditions had worsened, and the boy had grown into a young man, while I had become his devoted companion.

Inseparable, joined by love, we also shared the fierce conviction that there was no choice but to fight against the aggressors. Our anger over injustice spilled out and was directed against Grandmother. The ensuing arguments bordered on disrespect.

I bore him two children - a boy and a girl. But even the blessings of family were not enough to calm the waters of discontent and disagreement; and our iron-clad conviction remained - that aggression must be met with aggression.

A small group of young warriors met privately, repeatedly. When it became clear that my man was about to leave the village to join with the other braves who chose to fight on their own, I insisted I would not be left behind. No longer trusting Grandmother, Mother, or Father, I bundled up my babies and fled to another village, where I entrusted my children's care to a friend.

I and the warriors fought hard; but turning back the rising tide of Europeans was, of course, impossible. Sacrifice had only made our small band more self-righteous, and although hostility had carried us through the difficult struggle, the many murders we committed had cast our fate.

In the end, my man and I used what little strength we had left to make our way home. Wounded and slowly dying, we crawled the last bit of distance into the village to find our children. Our small daughter, too young to understand, reached out with her hand to touch and taste our blood, while our son, sobbing, slapped her hand away, and then embraced his sister as we, their parents, died.

A good metaphor for life is that it is a "play", and we are all actors with specific parts assigned to us. Some of my present-day family — David, Krystal, and I — and some of Dr. London's present-day family — Judy, Sadie, and he — were joined together in that Indian life. And although the script has changed, and the parts are very different now, we are together again in this life.

What we make of this opportunity is up to us.

Recently, during a very difficult time, and being nearly beside myself with worry, I prepared to go into town. I was all wrapped up in "problem solving" and was preparing to go on a "mission." But before I left the house, I sat down to have a quick cup of coffee. Imagine my surprise when several "spirits" joined me at the table! Dr. London's sister, parents, and grandparents, along with my aunt, my mother and my grandmother, had arrived in full force to support me. And I couldn't help but wonder if they'd stopped along the way at McDonald's since they all seemed to have their own cups of coffee in hand!

When I got into my car, I glanced behind me, and lo and behold, Judy, Sadie and my aunt (who had run with Geronimo and me in a past life), were right there in the back seat, prepared to go with me as further support! As I drove out of the yard, I noticed Hildegard standing in the yard, waving to me.

I realize this may all sound like fantasy, but what does it really matter if in the end it helps me feel as though I am always surrounded by caring and supportive "family." Never before had this particular group of spirits come together at the same time to help me. But, for me, this was an "extreme emergency." Apparently they understood my dire need.

Comforted by their presence, I drove into town, calm and steady.

I believe that my story, my attachment to the past and to the American Indian struggle, has determined the challenges I face in this present life. The sins of the fathers and mothers are passed on to their sons and daughters. I am my own ancestor. My sin from that other life is passed on to me in this life. If I am to heal myself, I must also heal my line; and that line leads right back to who I was and what I did in the past.

Many people believe that family comes first. But who exactly are the members of my family? Is my friend in this life — the one who was my child in a past life — still a part of my family now? For me, the answer is a resounding yes!

Everything is connected: the past, the present, and the future - who we once were, who we are today, and who we will be tomorrow. Everything we do matters! We have a chance to make things right in this life. And walking the labyrinth, moving into a meditative state and connecting with all that is — as well as learning what our "stories" are — can help us with our healing.

16 - Famous guests

There have been too many instances throughout the years when people have had a good laugh at Shirley MacLaine (and others like her) because of her belief in reincarnation. The laughter is sometimes accompanied by a rolling of the eyes. It takes a bit of courage to stand your ground when you become the butt of jokes; and credibility can be lost instantly when someone who is "psychic" claims to have had contact with a famous personality who is no longer living. But the plain fact is that there really are times when a well-known entity comes through with a message. Make of it what you will, but I have had such "visitations."

One occurred right after I met Dr. London. I "saw" Sigmund Freud. And his message was very clear: Dr. London's family would not stand behind him when research took him away from the traditional and into the revolutionary. At the time, I also understood that it would be good for me to offer up my support.

Another "famous" visitation happened recently. Haile Selassie, of Ethiopia, appeared to me. I had greatly admired him ever since I first learned who he was and what his accomplishments were way back when I was not yet out of my teens. He also had a message for Dr. London - and it had to do with healing and karma. One thing I found oddly interesting was that the man was dressed in a blue sport coat, which seemed not at all how I always imagined him dressing. But then, soon afterward, I happened to see a photograph in which he was, indeed, in a blue sport coat! I always enjoy the little details which, for me, offer some validation to my visions!

17 - Today

Although I have not been restored to perfect health, I am grateful for the fact that I have experienced many gains. In particular, the terrible fatigue I once dealt with is gone, and I no longer require daytime naps. I use a walker or canes to get around, but sensation has returned to my whole body; the numbness which for years traveled throughout my legs and body is gone, and I have begun to lift my left leg more than before. But, for me, the greatest gift of healing truly is the lack of debilitating fatigue which plagued me for decades. Now, I can get up early, put in my hours of meditation, receive visitors for spiritual counseling, have dinner with my husband, and not feel tired. So, here I am in my early sixties having far more energy than I had at forty. And in my book, that truly is a healing.

Peace, love and joy

Sara

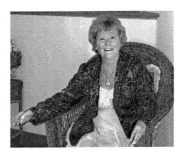

Acknowledgments

My family, husband David, son Steven, daughter Kristal and grandchildren. Thanks for all the love and support.

My friend, June Sager, thanks for listening, listening, and listening.

My friend, Patty McMahon, thanks for all the hours talking and your work organizing my rambling which resulted in this book, *Sara's Story*.

Paul Eagle for the book layout and illustrations.

And I also thank Wayne P. London, M.D., who showed me a path of healing that changed the course of my life.

Medical Epilogue

By Wayne P. London, M.D.

©2010   Brattleboro, VT

It seems to me that Western science and Eastern philosophy can join together to create a really complete and full-fledged human being. It is only in this way that man will emerge strengthened from his condition and become whole. What in fact interests me is what is beyond matter and awareness, what really is important, and what makes us what we are.

- HH the Dalai Lama

In describing the moment in time to which a divined hexagram refers, Richard Wilhelm writes in the introduction to his translation of The Book of Changes: "... every event in the visible world is the effect of an 'image', that is, of an idea in the unseen world. Accordingly, everything that happens on earth is only a reproduction, as it were, of an event in a world beyond our sense perception; as regards its occurrence in time, it is later than the suprasensible event.

– R.L. Wing, *I Ching Workbook*

Attachment is our greatest self-cruelty.

-Sujata

Introduction

Sara's story is an invitation to consider disease as "dis-ease." When we add a hyphen to the word disease, we can perhaps see more clearly that a diseased condition is a condition of being "not at ease." From dis-ease, one may then return to "ease." In

> **Sara's dis-ease indicated that Sara was not at ease.**

Sara's case, the auto-immune disease of multiple sclerosis (M.S.) was a clear sign of "dis-ease." The standard medical approach to M.S. is to prescribe medications to fight the physical symptoms. But treating disease this way seems a shortsighted and incomplete view. Instead of attacking the symptoms of a problem, can we seek to fix the problem itself?

Can we consider <u>how</u> Sara was "not at ease"? Disease certainly exists in the physical body. But it may also involve a problem throughout a person's being. Dis-ease may also exist in the metaphysical ("beyond physical") realms of spirituality and belief. So while Sara's problem appeared in her physical body as M.S., it also had metaphysical and spiritual aspects. Her story tells of her treatment as a whole being through MASH therapies.

MASH stands for Metaphysical and Spiritual Healing. It's a spiritual approach to living, to biology, to dis-ease and to healing, where health and healing mean wholeness. MASH assumes that people are spirit in a physical body, and that people have souls and metaphysical experiences that transcend physical space and time. Events in the physical world, including relationships and diseases, are opportunities for advancement or evolution of the soul.

Diseases may be healing crises — episodes that may be considered problematic by the person experiencing them, but that also contain clues for further growth and evolution of the soul. Dis-ease may in fact contain the seeds of improved ease. Sara's progress with her multiple sclerosis is an excellent case study of how MASH treats the whole being — physical, spiritual, individual, universal, past, present and future.

Western medicine's view of auto-immune diseases

Background

Multiple sclerosis is an auto-immune disease, which is a condition where a person's immune system attacks his or her own body as if the body were a foreign "other" to be destroyed. Basically, the body's defense system fights the body that houses it — a sort of internal war. Of course, the body's immune system is normally supposed to attack outside invaders, such as viruses (colds, flu) or bacteria (traveler's diarrhea, tuberculosis). But with an auto-immune disease, this powerful system starts destroying the body itself in a "mistaken" response. There are more than 80 of these diseases,[1] including multiple sclerosis, Type I diabetes, lupus and rheumatoid arthritis (RA). In the case of Type I diabetes, the immune system attacks the cells of the pancreas, impairing the body's ability to use blood glucose (fuel for the body's cells). In the case of RA, the joints are affected. Lupus may affect joints or an organ or system of the body.

In the case of M.S., the attack is on the nervous system. Specifically, with M.S., the immune system attacks the myelin that sheathes and protects the nerves, particularly in the brain, spinal cord and/or optic nerves. As this protective coating becomes damaged and scarred, nerve impulses can no longer travel properly or at all. Symptoms of M.S. include numbness, tremors, problems with balance and coordination, pain, memory problems, loss of bladder or bowel control, inability to walk, vision problems, strong feelings of fatigue—and many more difficulties.[2] M.S. typically comes in episodes or attacks. The person may recover between episodes, but as the immune system continues to do its "mistaken" job, the degeneration of the nerves continues and the person loses more and more function.

The National Multiple Sclerosis Society divides M.S. experiences into 4 courses—a person may have relapses followed by remissions, may have slow degeneration with some pauses, may have first relapses and remissions and then slow degeneration, or may have steady degeneration with no remissions. Each experience is different and may be mild, extreme or in between.[3]

Treatment

Western medicine knows no cure for M.S. (or other auto-immune diseases), but instead aims to treat symptoms and control progress of the disease. Certain powerful drugs (such as interferons) may be prescribed to decrease the disease activity.[4] Steroids may be prescribed to lessen the inflammation that characterizes attacks. Antidepressants may be prescribed for the mental effects of disease. Medications may also be prescribed for the urinary incontinence, for the fatigue, for the muscle spasms, and for the other symptoms that accompany M.S.. Rehabilitation therapies are encouraged if possible, such as physical therapy, speech therapy and occupational therapy. People with M.S. may also rely on wheelchairs, walkers and other assistive devices. Sara Willis uses a walker or canes, for example.

Unfortunately, the drugs Western medicine uses to combat the body's own immune system are very powerful (some are also used for fighting cancer) and can have serious side effects. For example, interferons are a class of drugs that are "immunomodulators" or "biologic response modifiers." Their job is to sideline how the body's natural defenses work. Usually injected, interferons have a stunning range of side effects: joint pain, toothache, strange dreams, hair loss, tingling, incontinence, impotence, constipation, confusion and crossed eyes are just a few. These drugs also carry "important warnings" (a bit like a pack of cigarettes) for more serious and rare side effects like suicidal thoughts, hallucinations and difficulty breathing. Other drugs used for auto-immune disease are so powerful that their side effects include heart damage, kidney failure and cancer. Natalizumab is so risky that users must register for a monitoring program to keep track of their health while they take the drug. How bad must the symptoms be if the treatment for them causes cancer? Why not stop sledge-hammering the symptoms and look at the whole, intricate problem from a holistic level? Sara tried various medications and treatments, but she found "the ones I tried did not help; and those I refused to try didn't appear to be helping anyone else suffering from multiple sclerosis" (Chapter 9).

MASH's holistic perspective on autoimmune disease

Background

The MASH approach adds to Western medicine's understanding of auto-immune disease as a condition in which the immune system attacks the body. MASH sees auto-immune disease as an attack on the <u>whole</u> self — both physical and metaphysical. An auto-immune disease involves something going awry with how the immune system distinguishes self from not-self. MASH gives thought to the basic question of why the immune system is attacking the self. Why would a person's immune system target part of his or her body for destruction? Might the reason differ between individuals? Is there a way to diagnose or identify this reason? How can we offer whole-self holistic treatment?

> **An autoimmune disease is the physiological equivalent of friendly fire.**

The following diagram (Figure 1) helps explain the MASH view of "dis-ease," and of auto-immune diseases in particular.

The Immune System: Self--Not-Self / Kill--Not Kill; In--Not-In / Belong--Not-Belong

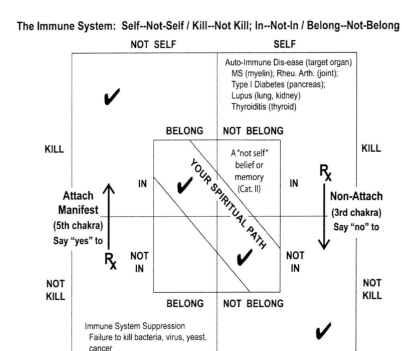

Figure 1. The Immune System

Take a look at the labels on the large, outer boxes in this grid. The left-hand column represents "not self" (things foreign to the person's body or spirit). The right-hand column represents "self" (things that belong in the person's body or spirit). The top row represents "kill" (the natural action of the immune system to destroy problems) and the bottom row represents "not kill" (the immune system does not act). Check marks in the upper left and lower right boxes mark the usual action of the immune system. That is, it is normal and preferred for the immune system to Kill Not-Self (such as fighting off a cold or flu virus that has invaded the body) — the upper left box. It is normal and preferred for the immune system to Not Kill Self (such as taking no destructive action against the person's own organs and systems) — the bottom right box. But look at the upper right box. This represents cases where the immune system acts to Kill Self. The immune system attacks the person's own body — the definition of auto-immune disease.

As described above, auto-immune disease often targets a specific organ or system. Myelin is the target organ in multiple sclerosis; the islet cells of the pancreas in Type 1 insulin dependent diabetes; the joints in rheumatoid arthritis; the lungs, kidney and other organs in lupus; the connective tissue in scleroderma; and the thyroid gland in Hashimoto's thyroiditis. In short, the person's immune system, meant to defend against germs and not-self, instead directs its fury against the person's own tissues — self. It's the physiological equivalent of friendly fire. Why would the immune system make this "mistake"? The next diagram (Figure 2), helps explain.

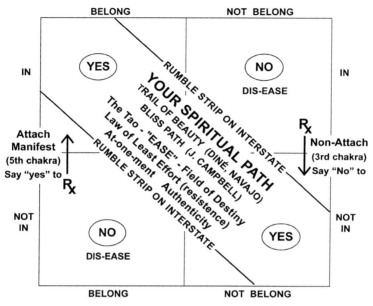

Figure 2: Spiritual Path

Here, instead of "Self/Not-Self" and "Kill/Not Kill," the categories are "Belong/Not Belong" (left and right columns) and "In/Not In" (top and bottom rows). Instead of depicting the immune system's action, this grid shows one's spiritual path and possible areas of holistic "dis-ease." The spiritual path runs from the top left corner to the bottom right. At the top left, "Belong-In" means that the things that belong in your life are in fact in your life. You're on your spiritual path. At the bottom right, "Not Belong-Not In" means that things that don't belong in your life are not in your life. Again, you're on your spiritual path here. The Spiritual Path goes by many names: The Tao, Ease,

Field of Destiny, At-one-ment (re-punctuating atonement), authenticity, and so forth.

But what happens if you somehow stray from this path? One sign of getting off course is encountering resistance: physical, social or spiritual problems, for example. These problems are the "rumble strip" — that noisy, bumpy signal that one is veering off the road. Problems "on the edge" include dis-ease, both physical and metaphysical. You stray into not having things in your life that belong there, or having things in your life that do not belong. These are states of "dis-ease." Going back to Figure 1, you'll see that the inside box is a thumbnail of Figure 2. When one is in the area of Not Belong being In the body, one is in the realm of auto-immune disease — the realm of Kill Self. In other words, the Not Belong/In quadrant matches up with the Kill Self quadrant, the area of auto-immune disease. MASH seeks to define what does not belong. When we do that, we can stop the Kill Self reaction.

> **An autoimmune disease suggests something IN your life that does NOT BELONG.**

Healing Strategy

Let's review how Western medicine treats auto-immune disease. Western medicine finds that the immune system is making a mistake and killing self. So the treatments try to kill (or suppress or

> **The Western approach to auto-immune disease is that the immune system is killing us, so let's kill it.**

modulate) the immune system so it will no longer wreak havoc in the body. The Western approach to auto-immune disease is that the immune system is killing us, so let's kill it. As mentioned, many autoimmune dis-eases are treated with cancer drugs or steroids. Unfortunately, the effects of these drugs can be quite severe. The underlying causes of dis-ease are not addressed or even understood. Little progress is made in figuring out why the immune system is attacking the self. MASH believes this approach is not working.

By contrast, MASH therapies don't destroy the village in order to save it. MASH believes that the immune system is not making a mistake, but doing its job correctly. It seems complicated and destructive to try to counter the body's own powerful and natural fighting force, the immune system, with outside fighting forces, particularly

> **By contrast, MASH therapies don't destroy the village in order to save it.**

hard-core (and seriously expensive) pharmaceuticals. A simpler and clearer approach is to take the immune system's message at face value. When the immune system is fighting self, we can ask "What do you have in your life that does not belong there? What is putting you in the Kill Self quadrant?" MASH follows the Law of Least Effort here.

According to Deepak Chopra's The Seven Spiritual Laws of Success,[6] the Law of Least Effort first involves accepting the intelligence of nature (in this case, accepting that the immune system is acting as it should). Second, it involves responding to each problem or experience as an opportunity to learn and grow, even if that thing would seem negative to most people. Third, it involves not fighting for or even adhering to a certain point of view. Instead, remaining open can make it easier to accept new approaches or new paths (or new healing techniques!) that may turn out to be essential on one's life journey. Sara was certainly open to alternative techniques, including exploring ideas of reincarnation.

The Two Steps to Healing: Identify and Non-Attach

After accepting that Sara's immune system's attacks have some purpose (rather than being a random, mistaken action), MASH must diagnose her metaphysical and spiritual issues in order to work toward healing. Another law, the Law of Karma, comes into play.[7] Karma can be explained simply as "what goes around comes around." If a person takes an action or has an experience that needs to be healed or "closed," his or her self will continue to experience the effects of that action or experience until closure or retribution is attained.

Karma can transcend human lifetimes, staying in the fields of space and time until it is addressed and healed. The karma of Sara's self showed up in her body as MS—it "came back around" in her current lifetime. MASH finds that the immune system is a karma memory system that responds to memories or

> **Two quotes by Yogi Berra are relevant: "It's *deja vu* all over again," and "You can observe a lot just by watching."**

learned experiences. So we must consider whether someone with an auto-immune disease has a memory in their life that does not belong. Is that Not-self memory being manifested on a part of their body—or even attaching to a specific organ or system of the body? If there is such a memory and attachment, the body's immune system may well try to fight off that not-self by fighting the target system or organ. Different themes of not-self manifest on different parts of the body. For Sara, her MS—an auto-immune disease with themes of movement—told her she must fix some karma that involved movement or action.

The two step MASH healing strategy is to (1) identify the stuck memory/story/karma, and (2) have the person or group non-attach to the stuck memory/story through ritual and chakra work. For Step 1, identifying, we look for what is in a person's life but does not belong. For Sara's MS, we ask: what is the not-self memory that is resonating with her myelin? Generally, a not-self memory could be a prior role, a prior experience or a prior group or cultural issue. Two quotes by Yogi Berra are relevant: "It's *deja vu* all over again," and "You can observe a lot just by watching." The person's dis-ease is a repetition of the memory or the story in their current lifetime, and identifying that story is, as Sara puts it, "one of the keys to healing the present (as well as the past)" (Chapter 14). What can we observe about the pattern of Sara's dis-ease experience?

One hint for finding Sara's not-self memory is that MS is a clear-cut warrior disease. As an archetype, the warrior is a person of action, of movement, of singular devotion to the mission. A disease that affects movement like MS does points to karma that is warrior-related. Sara was well aware of her "determination to be strong and capable," to fight and to do right however she could (Chapter 3). MASH finds that warrior memories/karma/experiences manifest across time and space in a certain cycle and in a certain proportion.

That cycle involves Phi (a.k.a., the Divine Proportion or Golden Mean, symbolized by the Greek letter *phi*, Φ) and what we call the "Semper Phi Warrior Sequence." The sequence is: 0, 4, 4, 8, 12, 20, 32, 52, 84, 136, 220, etc. Each term in the sequence is the sum of the preceding two terms. The Semper Phi Warrior Sequence can be used as a template for seeing patterns and identifying significant warrior events or memories. For example, if we assign one particular year to be 0 and then look at the sequence going back in time (what happened 4 years before? 8 years before? 12 years before? and so forth) it can help us find historical sources of karma/memories.

MASH applied the Semper Phi Warrior Sequence to Sara's current lifetime and found the year 1863 to be of significance. Taking Sara's birth year, 1947, and subtracting the sequence numbers one by one, the number 84 was particularly resonant. 1947 minus 84 is 1863. 1863 was the middle of the Civil War and a time of great unrest in America. It was also the time of the "Indian Wars" west of Mississippi, particularly the Apache Campaigns and the military career of the man called Geronimo. And indeed, Sara experienced strong identification with Geronimo and the Apache.

Sara had a fierce attachment to those Native American warrior events. Even as a child, she noted "I could not watch Westerns on television because my connection was to the Indians, not the cowboys. And

> *Attachment is our greatest self-cruelty.*
> **- Sujata**

as I learned more, I was not merely sympathetic; I was outraged" (Chapter 2). She also felt "deepening anger" over the treatment of the Apaches (Chapter 3). Late in the 20th century, Sara was still fighting the story of Geronimo and knew she was "fiercely attached" to that story. In fact, that war and that memory was showing up in her body as dis-ease, as MS.

To put herself back on her spiritual path, Sara needed to follow her bliss and steer away from the "rumble strip" that included violent, karmic memories. Sara's immune system recognized her fierce attachment to these memories as NOT SELF. The MASH

> **Sara's immune system recognized her fierce attachment to these memories as NOT SELF.**

prescription for her was that she must non-attach from the not-self memory that her body was fighting. First, there are many ways to do this, but having the intent to do it is essential. The Law of Attraction says that you are what you think — whether your thoughts are positive or negative, of love or of fear, those thoughts are what you will become.[8] For Sara, she had to detach from her repeated thoughts and visions and her intense anger about the Apache experience.

Being attached to the memory of a prior group warrior experience from the 1860's involving the Apaches and the Geronimo period did not belong in her current 20th century life. Her immune system recognized that memory as "not- self" and tried to do its job by attacking her myelin.

Sara's non-attaching process happened over a 3-month period of learning, absorbing, considering, crying, cleansing and releasing. Her husband gave her books on Native Americans that were key in uncovering her karma, doing her "proper grieving" and then letting go. By reading and crying and reading and crying, she was able to release that which did not belong in her life and start finding her "authentic self" (Chapter 11). She learned to speak and live her own truth. She learned to get back onto her spiritual path. And she found this work effective against her M.S.. Sensation has returned to her body, and numbness lifted. She writes that "the greatest gift of healing truly is the lack of debilitating fatigue which plagued me for decades" (Chapter 17). She did all this without drugs and without the phenomenal expense and worrisome risks of Western medicine.

Conclusion

Sara did not have an MRI or other diagnostic scan before or after her metaphysical and spiritual healing process. Therefore we cannot offer the evidence of healing that Western medicine might expect. Sara's story is one of spiritual tradition, and MASH offers its own effective evaluation tools and processes. The Geronimo/warrior story "put out the fire" of the disease in Sara's body. Sara is still debilitated – putting out the fire is not the same as rebuilding the house – and there could be more to her healing process. But when she non-attached to that prior group warrior experience by reading books about that time and grieving over those events with mindful attention and intention – the not-self stopped resonating with her myelin. Her immune system backed off and her autoimmune "internal war" stopped. She has shown sustained partial recovery since that time.

Sara Willis is one fascinating and successful case study. But auto-immune diseases affect 5-8 percent of the U.S. population.[5] As of 2009, that is around 15.3 million to 24.6 million people. Patient advocacy groups often give much higher estimates, and there is evidence that the incidence of some of the auto-immune diseases is increasing. But for Sara and perhaps for others, autoimmune disease could be a gift. Sara got a sign she was off her spiritual path, with warrior and "kill" motivations. Her true direction was not this violent one at all. She was equipped to be a healer and a seer. In her current lifetime she has been able to unravel the tangle of karma that was hurting her, and to organize her healing energies and abilities in a clear and helpful way. She has even built a healing labyrinth near her home, a legacy for the future.

Medical Epilogue sources:

1) nlm.nih.gov/medlineplus/autoimmunediseases.html
2) nlm.nih.gov/medlineplus/ency/article/000737.htm
3) nationalmssociety.org/about-multiple-sclerosis/
   what-is-ms
4) nationalmssociety.org/about-multiple-
   sclerosis/treatments
5) www3.niaid.nih.gov/topics/autoimmune
6) Chopra, Deepak, The Seven Spiritual Laws of Success,
   San Rafael, CA, Amber-Allen Publishing & New
   World Library, 1994, pp. 53-64: the Law of Least Effort
7) ibid., pp. 37-50: the Law of Karma.
8) ibid., pp. 65-80: the Law of Intention and Desire.

Addendum to the Medical Epilogue

By Wayne P. London, M.D.
©2010 Brattleboro, VT

We shall require a substantially new manner of thinking if humanity is to survive.

- Albert Einstein

Not only are we connected in the physical to all things in the present, but we are also connected to our past and future. We need to bring our indigenous knowledge forward as a means for our survival. This does not mean we go back to living as we did in the past, it means we bring forward our ancestor's way of thought and actions. We must change our way of thought and actions if we are going to survive.

- Ella Mulford, a member of the Diné (Navajo) Nation

Since the preparation of this Medical Epilogue to *Sara's Story*, material on the Field or the Body Field has appeared (viz. *The Living Matrix,* thelivingmatrixmovie.com). This material provides a context for Sara's healing odyssey and the MASH approach to auto immune dis-eases. The two basic premises of the Field or Body Field approach to healing as described in *The Living Matrix* are:

1) **Health or Ease is accessing "authentic" information from the Body Field that programs or directs the physical body including the immune system.** This "authentic" information is a "signal" that your body as a receptor receives or re-takes. In the MASH formulation, this "authentic" information or signal would be what <u>belongs</u> in your life.

2) **Dis-ease is accessing a "defective or scrambled", i.e. non-authentic, information or signal.** In the MASH formulation, this would be what does <u>not belong</u> in your life.

The field, or body field, of *The Living Matrix* also corresponds to the "field" of Ancient Chinese wisdom.

Sara's intense attachment to the Apache Native American warrior events that occurred in the phi proportion circa 84 years before she was born would be non-authentic information that was recognized by her immune system.

From the point of view of the Body Field as described in *The Living Matrix*, the MASH approach to auto immune dis-eases is attachment to defective or scrambled information that is detected by the immune system. The healing solution is non-attachment to this defective information or signal.

Sara's healing odyssey would be an example of the Body Field approach to health, wholeness and Ease as described in *The Living Matrix*.

Links between "images" or the "field of images" of ancient Chinese wisdom, the Field or the Body Field as described in *The Living Matrix* and Sara's spiritual path and her auto immune dis-ease are shown in Figure 3.

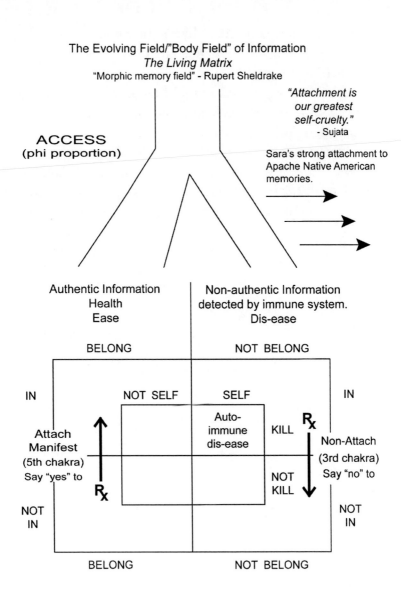

Figure 3. Sara's M.S. and *The Living Matrix*

Contact Sara

Book ordering and additional information can be found online at **SaraWillis.org**.